# Contents

## INTRODUCTION

Lymphedema is very common and serious condition that affects millions of individuals. While there is no consistency in the data of the overall incidence of lymphedema in the United States, it is estimated that at least 3 million Americans are affected by this condition.

Lymphedema is classified as either primary or secondary. Primary lymphedema is caused by congenital malformations of the lymphatic system and usually affects the lower extremities. It may be present at birth, but more often develops later in life, often in puberty or during pregnancy.

Secondary lymphedema is much more common; most patients in the western hemisphere develop lymphedema after surgery and/or radiation therapy for various cancers (breast, uterus, prostate, bladder, lymphoma, and melanoma). Other patients develop lymphedema after trauma or deep vein thrombosis. In certain countries, parasites (filariasis) account for millions of cases of lymphedema. Its cosmetic deformities are difficult to hide, and complications, such as fibrosis, cellulitis, lymphangitis, lymphorrhea, etc. do occur frequently. Lymphedema may be present in the extremities, trunk, head and neck, abdomen, the external genitalia as well as in inner organs; its onset is gradual in some patients and sudden in others.

The focus of this is to discuss the role of nutrition as an additional approach to manage lymphedema effectively.

# Chapter One

## What is Lymphedema?

Lymphedema is impaired flow of the lymphatic system that causes swollen extremities. Lymphedema is a condition that results from impaired flow of the lymphatic system.

Symptoms of lymphedema include swelling in one or more extremities. The swelling may range from mild to severe and disfiguring.

Primary lymphedema is present at birth; secondary lymphedema develops as a result of damage to or dysfunction of the lymphatic system. Breast cancer treatment is the most common cause of lymphedema in the U.S.

While there is no cure for lymphedema, compression treatments and physical therapy may help reduce the swelling and discomfort.

Lymphedema is a chronic, debilitating condition in which excess fluid called lymph collects in tissues and causes swelling (edema) in them. Lymphedema symptoms include swelling of the limbs, cracked and thickening skin, and secondary bacterial or fungal infections.

In addition to the swelling, other symptoms can include:

• Warmth, redness, or itching

• Tingling or burning pains

- Fever and chills

- Decreased flexibility in the joints

- Aching, pain, and fullness in the affected area

- Skin rash

- Suppressed immune function in affected area

The lymphatic system is a network of specialized vessels (lymph vessels) throughout the body whose purpose is to collect excess lymph fluid with proteins, lipids, and waste products from the tissues. This fluid is then carried to the lymph nodes, which filter waste products and contain infection-fighting cells called lymphocytes. The excess fluid in the lymph vessels is eventually returned to the bloodstream. When the lymph vessels are blocked or unable to carry lymph fluid away from the tissues, localized swelling (lymphedema) is the result.

Lymphedema most often affects a single arm or leg, but in uncommon situations both limbs are affected.

Primary lymphedema is the result of an anatomical abnormality of the lymph vessels and is a rare, inherited condition.

Secondary lymphedema results from an identifiable damage to or obstruction of normally-functioning lymph vessels and nodes.

Worldwide, lymphedema is most commonly caused by filariasis (a parasite infection), but in the U.S., lymphedema most commonly occurs in women who have had breast cancer surgery, particularly when followed by radiation treatment.

Mild lymphedema first may be noticed as a feeling of heaviness, tingling, tightness, warmth, or shooting pains in the affected extremity. These symptoms may be present before there is obvious swelling of an arm or leg. Other signs and symptoms of early or mild lymphedema include:

• a decreased ability to see or feel the veins or tendons in the extremities,

• tightness of jewelry or clothing,

• redness of the skin,

• asymmetrical appearance of the extremities,

• tightness or reduced flexibility in the joints, and

• Slight puffiness of the skin.

As lymphedema progresses to a more moderate to severe state, the swelling of the involved extremity becomes more pronounced. The other symptoms mentioned above also persist with moderate or severe lymphedema.

Primary lymphedema is an abnormality of an individual's lymphatic system and is generally present at birth, although symptoms may not become apparent until later in life. Depending upon the age at which symptoms develop, three forms of primary lymphedema have been described. Most primary lymphedema occurs without any known family history of the condition.

Congenital lymphedema is evident at birth, is more common in females, and accounts for about 10-25% of all cases of primary lymphedema. A subgroup of people with congenital lymphedema has a genetic inheritance (in medical genetics termed "familial sex-linked pattern"), which is termed Milroy disease.

Lymphedema praecox is the most common form of primary lymphedema. It is defined as lymphedema that becomes apparent after birth and before age 35 years and symptoms most often develop during puberty. Lymphedema praecox is four times more common in females than in males.

Primary lymphedema that becomes evident after 35 years of age is known as Meige disease or lymphedema tarda. It is less common than congenital lymphedema and lymphedema praecox.


**Secondary lymphedema causes**

Secondary lymphedema develops when a normally-functioning lymphatic system is blocked or damaged. In the U.S., breast cancer surgery, particularly when combined with radiation treatment, is the most common cause. This results in one-sided (unilateral) lymphedema of the arm. Any type of surgical procedure that requires removal of regional lymph nodes or lymph vessels can potentially cause lymphedema. Surgical procedures that have been associated with lymphedema include vein stripping, lipectomy, burn scar excision, and peripheral vascular surgery.

Damage to lymph nodes and lymph vessels, leading to lymphedema, can also occur due to trauma, burns, radiation, infections, or compression or invasion of lymph nodes by tumors.

Worldwide, however, filariasis is the most common cause of lymphedema. Filariasis is the direct infestation of lymph nodes by the parasite Wuchereria bancrofti. The disease is spread among persons by mosquitoes, and affects millions of people in the tropics and subtropics of Asia, Africa, Western Pacific, and parts of Central and South America. Infestation by the parasite damages the lymph system, leading to swelling in the arms, breasts, legs, and, for men, the genital area. The entire leg, arm, or genital area may swell to several times its normal size. Also, the swelling and the decreased function of the lymph system make it difficult for the body to fight infections. Lymphatic filariasis is a leading cause of permanent disability in the world.

## What are possible treatments for lymphedema?

There is no cure for lymphedema. Treatments are designed to reduce the swelling and control discomfort and other symptoms.

Compression treatments can help reduce swelling and prevent scarring and other complications. Examples of compression treatments are:

• Elastic sleeves or stockings: These must fit properly and provide gradual compression from the end of the extremity toward the trunk.

• Bandages: Bandages that are wrapped more tightly around the end of the extremity and wrapped more loosely toward the trunk, to encourage lymph flow out of the extremity toward the center of the body.

• Pneumatic compression devices: These are sleeves or stockings connected to a pump that provides sequential compression from the end of the extremity toward the body. These may be used in the clinic or in the home and are useful in preventing long-term scarring, but they cannot be used in all individuals, such as those with congestive heart failure, deep venous thrombosis, or certain infections.

• Manual compression: Massage techniques, known as manual lymph drainage, can be useful for some people with lymphedema.

• Exercises: Exercises that lightly contract and stimulate arm or leg muscles may be prescribed by the doctor or physical therapist to help stimulate lymph flow.

Surgical treatments for lymphedema are used to remove excess fluid and tissue in severe cases, but no surgical treatment is able to cure lymphedema.

Infections of skin and tissues associated with lymphedema must be promptly and effectively treated with appropriate antibiotics to avoid spread to the bloodstream (sepsis). Patients affected by lymphedema must constantly monitor for infection of the affected area. In affected areas of the world, the drug diethylcarbamazine is used to treat filariasis.

## What are complications of lymphedema? Can lymphedema be fatal?

As noted before, secondary infections of the skin and underlying tissues can complicate lymphedema. Inflammation of the skin and connective tissues, known as cellulitis, and inflammation of the lymphatic vessels (lymphangitis) are common complications of lymphedema. Deep venous thrombosis (formation of blood clots in the deeper veins) is also a known complication of lymphedema. Impairment of functioning in the affected area and cosmetic issues are further complications of lymphedema.

Those who have had chronic, long-term lymphedema for more than 10 years have a 10% chance of developing a cancer of the lymphatic vessels known as lymphangiosarcoma. The cancer begins as a reddish or purplish lump visible on the skin and spreads rapidly. This is an aggressive cancer that is treated by amputation of the affected limb. Even with treatment, the prognosis is poor, with less than 10% of patients surviving after 5 years.

## Can lymphedema be prevented?

Primary lymphedema cannot be prevented, but measures can be taken to reduce the risk of developing lymphedema if one is at risk for secondary lymphedema, such as after cancer surgery or radiation treatment.

The following steps may help reduce the risk of developing lymphedema in those at risk for secondary lymphedema:

• Keep the affected arm or leg elevated above the level of the heart, when possible.

• Avoid tight or constricting garments or jewelry (also avoid the use of blood pressure cuffs on an affected arm).

• Do not apply a heating pad to the affected area or use hot tubs, steam baths, etc.

• Keep the body adequately hydrated.

• Avoid heavy lifting and forceful activity with the affected limb; but normal, light activity is encouraged.

• Do not carry a heavy purse on an affected arm.

• Practice thorough and careful skin hygiene.

• Avoid insect bites and sunburns.

## What is the prognosis for lymphedema? Is lymphedema curable?

Lymphedema cannot be cured, but compression treatments and preventive measures for those at risk for secondary lymphedema can help minimize swelling and associated symptoms. As mentioned above, chronic, long-term edema that persists for many years is associated with an increased risk of developing a rare cancer, lymphangiosarcoma.

## Where can one get help and support for lymphedema?

Many hospitals and treatment centers have support groups for people dealing with specific chronic conditions. Health care professionals may be able to recommend a local support group for those with lymphedema.

The National Lymphedema Network (NLN) is a non-profit organization founded in 1988 to provide education and guidance to lymphedema patients, health care professionals, and the general public by disseminating information on the prevention and management of primary and secondary lymphedema.

**Diuretics**

Diuretics promote excess fluid in the body to be excreted. Although diuretics may be beneficial in the short-term, and may be indicated in those cases when lymphedema is associated with systemic conditions (ascites, hydrothorax, protein-losing enteropathy), they may be harmful and contribute to the worsening of lymphedema-related symptoms if used long-term.

Here is why: Lymphedema is an abnormal accumulation of water and protein molecules in the body's soft tissues, which is caused by a dysfunction of the lymphatic system. Swelling (edema) other than lymphedema may be caused by a variety of conditions, such as congestive heart failure, renal diseases, or venous insufficiencies. These swellings do not contain a higher level of proteins in the accumulated fluid, and are defined as edemas.

Diuretics used for lymphedema are limited to remove the water content of the swelling, while the protein molecules remain in the soft tissues. The dehydration effect of diuretics causes a higher concentration of the protein mass in the edema fluid, which may cause the tissues to become more fibrotic and increase the potential for secondary inflammations. In addition, the remaining proteins characteristically draw more water to the swollen areas as soon as the diuretic loses its effectiveness and may cause the volume of the lymphedema to increase.

The 2009 Consensus Document (4) of the International Society of Lymphology states: "Diuretic agents are occasionally useful during the initial treatment phase of complete decongestive therapy (CDT). Long-term administration, however, is discouraged for its marginal benefits in treatment of peripheral lymphedema and potentially may induce fluid and electrolyte imbalance"

## What about Vitamins and other Supplements?

There are no vitamins, food supplements or herbs that have been proven to be effective in the reduction of lymphedema. In the United States, dietary supplements are regulated as food, not drugs. Pre-market approval by the Food and Drug Administration (FDA) are not required unless specific disease prevention or treatment claims are made. Because there is no requirement to review dietary supplements for manufacturing consistency, and no specific standards for dosage or purity exist, there may be considerable variation within the products marketed as dietary supplements.

However, individuals affected by lymphedema are often in need of additional vitamins and supplements, especially if they battle recurrent episodes of infections. To determine which supplements and vitamins are beneficial, patients should consult with their physicians and/or nutritional specialist.

# CHAPTER TWO

## Homemade Taco Seasoning Mix

"Much lower salt than pre-made. Salt can be omitted. Great with half ground buffalo and half ground turkey breast or whatever you prefer. Buy bulk spices and you can make 5-plus batches for under $1.00!! Increasing black pepper and adding optional ingredients will increase heat. Using mild or regular chili powder and omitting optional ingredients will reduce heat. To keep salt content low make sure chili powder does not contain salt."

**Ingredients**

5 m4 servings12 cals

- 2 teaspoons of hot chili powder

- 1 1/2 teaspoons of paprika

- 1 teaspoon of onion powder

- 1/2 teaspoon of sea salt

- 1/2 teaspoon of garlic powder

- 1/2 teaspoon of ground cumin

- 1/2 teaspoon of oregano

- 1/4 teaspoon of freshly ground black pepper, or to taste

- 1 pinch of cayenne pepper, or to taste (optional)

- 1 pinch of red pepper flakes, or to taste (optional)

- Add all ingredients to list

## Directions

1. Mix chili powder, paprika, onion powder, sea salt, garlic powder, cumin, oregano, and black pepper, cayenne pepper, and red pepper flakes in a bowl.

- Add to browning meat when meat is partially browned. After browned completely, add 1/2 to 1 cup water and cook down to blend flavors.

- Partner Tip

- Try using a Reynolds® slow cooker liner in your slow cooker for easier cleanup.

## Nutrition Facts

Per Serving: 12 calories; 0.5 g fat; 2.4 g carbohydrates;0.5 g protein; 0 mg cholesterol; 235 mg sodium. Full nutrition

**Recipe Summary**

Prep: 5 mins

Cook: 20 mins

Total: 40 mins

Additional: 15 mins

Servings: 8

Yield: 8 eggs

**Ingredients**

1 tablespoon of salt

¼ cup distilled white vinegar

6 cups water

8 eggs

**Directions**

Step 1

Combine the salt, vinegar, and water in a large pot, and bring to a boil over high heat. Add the eggs one at a time, being careful not to crack them. Reduce the heat to a gentle boil, and cook for 14 minutes.

Step 2

Once the eggs have cooked, remove them from the hot water, and place into a container of ice water or cold, running water. Cool completely, about 15 minutes. Store in the refrigerator up to 1 week.

**Nutrition Facts**

Per Serving:

72 calories; 5 g total fat; 186 mg cholesterol; 947 mg sodium. 0.4 g carbohydrates; 6.3 g protein; Full Nutrition

## Roasted Okra

**Recipe Summary**

Prep: 5 mins

Cook: 15 mins

Total: 20 mins

Servings: 3

**Ingredients**

18 fresh okra pods, sliced 1/3 inch thick

1 tablespoon of olive oil

2 teaspoons of kosher salt, or to taste

2 teaspoons of black pepper, or to taste

**Directions**

Step 1

Preheat an oven to 425 degrees F (220 degrees C).

Step 2

Arrange the okra slices in one layer on a foil lined cookie sheet. Drizzle with olive oil and sprinkle with salt and pepper. Bake in the preheated oven for 10 to 15 minutes.

**Nutrition Facts**

Per Serving:

65 calories; 4.6 g total fat; 0 mg cholesterol; 1286 mg sodium. 5.9 g carbohydrates; 1.6 g protein; Full Nutrition

## Spaghetti Sauce with Ground Beef

**Recipe Summary**

Prep: 15 mins

Cook: 1 hr 10 mins

Total: 1 hr 25 mins

Servings: 8

**Ingredients**

1 pound of ground beef

1 onion, chopped

4 cloves of garlic, minced

1 small green bell pepper, diced

1(28 ounce) can of diced tomatoes

1(16 ounce) can of tomato sauce

1(6 ounce) can of tomato paste

2 teaspoons of dried oregano

2 teaspoons of dried basil

1 teaspoon of salt

½ teaspoon of black pepper

**Directions**

Step 1

Combine ground beef, onion, garlic, and green pepper in a large saucepan. Cook and stir until meat is brown and vegetables are tender. Drain grease.

Step 2

Stir diced tomatoes, tomato sauce, and tomato paste into the pan. Season with oregano, basil, salt, and pepper. Simmer spaghetti sauce for 1 hour, stirring occasionally.

**Nutrition Facts**

Per Serving:

185 calories; 9.3 g total fat; 35 mg cholesterol; 931 mg sodium. 15 g carbohydrates; 12.4 g protein; Full Nutrition

## Roasted Asparagus Prosciutto and Egg

**Recipe Summary**

Prep: 15 mins

Cook: 25 mins

Total: 40 mins

Servings: 4

**Ingredients**

1 bunch of fresh asparagus, trimmed

1 tablespoon of extra-virgin olive oil

1 tablespoon of olive oil

2 ounces of minced prosciutto

Ground black pepper

1 teaspoon of distilled white vinegar

1 pinch of salt

4 eggs

½ lemon, zested and juiced

1 pinch of ground black pepper


**Directions**

Step 1

Preheat oven to 425 degrees F (220 degrees C). Place asparagus in a baking dish and drizzle with 1 tablespoon extra-virgin olive oil.

Step 2

Heat 1 tablespoon olive oil in a skillet over medium-low heat. Add prosciutto; cook, stirring, until golden and rendered, 3 to 4 minutes. Sprinkle prosciutto and oil over asparagus. Season with black pepper and toss to coat. Roast in the preheated oven for 10 minutes. Toss and return to oven until firm yet tender to the bite, 5 minutes.

Step 3

Fill a large saucepan with 2 to 3 inches of water and bring to a boil over high heat. Reduce heat to medium-low; pour in vinegar and pinch of salt. Crack an egg into a bowl then gently slip the egg into the water. Repeat with remaining eggs. Poach eggs until whites are firm and yolks have thickened but are not hard, 4 to 6 minutes. Remove eggs from water with a slotted spoon, dab on a kitchen towel to remove excess water, and then transfer to a warm plate.

Step 4

Drizzle asparagus with lemon juice. Transfer asparagus to plates, top with poached egg and pinch of lemon zest. Season with black pepper and serve.

**Nutrition Facts**

Per Serving:

199 calories; 15.7 g total fat; 175 mg cholesterol; 446 mg sodium. 5.1 g carbohydrates; 10.8 g protein; Full Nutrition

## Best Marinara Sauce

**Ingredients**

45 m

8 servings

151 cals

2 (14.5 ounce) cans stewed tomatoes 1 (6 ounce) can tomato paste 4 tablespoons chopped fresh parsley 1 clove garlic, minced 1 teaspoon dried oregano 1 teaspoon salt 1/4 teaspoon ground black pepper 6 tablespoons olive oil 1/3 cup finely diced onion 1/2 cup white wine Add all ingredients to list

**Directions**

Prep 15 m

Cook 30 m

Ready In 45 m

In a food processor place Italian tomatoes, tomato paste, chopped parsley, minced garlic, oregano, salt, and pepper. Blend until smooth.

In a large skillet over medium heat saute the finely chopped onion in olive oil for 2 minutes. Add the blended tomato sauce and white wine.

Simmer for 30 minutes, stirring occasionally.

**Nutrition Facts**

Per Serving: 151 calories; 10.5 g fat; 11.7 g carbohydrates; 2 g protein; 0 mg cholesterol; 685 mg sodium.


## Easy Herb Roasted Turkey

**Ingredients**

4 h 15 m

16 servings

597 cals

1 (12 pound) whole turkey 3/4 cup olive oil 2 tablespoons garlic powder 2 teaspoons dried basil 1

teaspoon ground sage 1 teaspoon salt 1/2 teaspoon black pepper 2 cups water Add all ingredients to list

## Directions

Preheat oven to 325 degrees F (165 degrees C). Clean turkey (discard giblets and organs), and place in a roasting pan with a lid.

In a small bowl, combine olive oil, garlic powder, dried basil, ground sage, salt, and black pepper. Using a basting brush, apply the mixture to the outside of the uncooked turkey. Pour water into the bottom of the roasting pan, and cover.

Bake for 3 to 3 1/2 hours, or until the internal temperature of the thickest part of the thigh measures 180 degrees F (82 degrees C). Remove bird from oven, and allow to stand for about 30 minutes before carving.

## Nutrition Facts

Per Serving: 597 calories; 33.7 g fat; 0.9 g carbohydrates; 68.2 g protein; 198 mg cholesterol; 311 mg sodium. Full nutrition

**Recipe Summary**

Prep: 15 mins

Total: 15 mins

Servings: 6

**Ingredients**

• 4 large ripe tomatoes, sliced 1/4 inch thick

• 1 pound of fresh mozzarella cheese, sliced 1/4 inch thick

• ⅓ cup of fresh basil leaves

• 3 tablespoons of extra virgin olive oil

• fine sea salt to taste

• freshly ground black pepper to taste

**Directions**

• Step 1

On a large platter, alternate and overlap the tomato slices, mozzarella cheese slices, and basil leaves. Drizzle with olive oil. Season with sea salt and pepper.

**Nutrition Facts**

Per Serving:

311 calories; 23.9 g total fat; 60 mg cholesterol; 627 mg sodium. 6.6 g carbohydrates; 17.9 g protein;

## Roast Sticky Chicken-Rotisserie Style

**Recipe Summary**

Prep: 10 mins

Cook: 5 hrs

Total: 9 hrs 10 mins

Additional: 4 hrs

Servings: 8

Yield: 2 whole (4 pound) chickens

**Ingredients**

4 teaspoons of salt

2 teaspoons of paprika

1 teaspoon of onion powder

1 teaspoon of dried thyme

1 teaspoon of white pepper

½ teaspoon of cayenne pepper

½ teaspoon of black pepper

½ teaspoon of garlic powder

2 onions, quartered

2(4 pound) whole chickens

**Directions**

Step 1

In a small bowl, mix together salt, paprika, onion powder, thyme, white pepper, black pepper, cayenne pepper, and garlic powder. Remove and discard giblets from chicken. Rinse chicken cavity, and pat dry with paper towel. Rub each chicken inside and out with spice mixture. Place 1 onion into the cavity of each chicken. Place chickens in a resalable bag or double wrap with plastic wrap. Refrigerate overnight or at least 4 to 6 hours.

Step 2

Preheat oven to 250 degrees F (120 degrees C).

Step 3

Place chickens in a roasting pan. Bake uncovered for 5 hours, to a minimum internal temperature of 180 degrees F (85 degrees C). Let the chickens stand for 10 minutes before carving.

**Nutrition Facts**

Per Serving:

586 calories; 34.3 g total fat; 194 mg cholesterol; 1351 mg sodium. 3.7 g carbohydrates; 61.7 g protein; Full Nutrition

## Simple Roasted Butternut Squash

**Recipe Summary**

Prep: 15 mins

Cook: 25 mins

Total: 40 mins

Servings: 4

**Ingredients**

1 butternut squash - peeled, seeded, and cut into 1-inch cubes

2 tablespoons of olive oil

2 cloves of garlic, minced

Salt and ground black pepper to taste

**Directions**

Step 1

Preheat oven to 400 degrees F (200 degrees C).

Step 2

Toss butternut squash with olive oil and garlic in a large bowl. Season with salt and black pepper. Arrange coated squash on a baking sheet.

Step 3

Roast in the preheated oven until squash is tender and lightly browned, 25 to 30 minutes.

**Nutrition Facts**

Per Serving:

177 calories; 7 g total fat; 0 mg cholesterol; 11 mg sodium. 30.3 g carbohydrates; 2.6 g protein; Full Nutrition

## Juicy Roasted Chicken

**Recipe Summary**

Prep: 10 mins

Cook: 1 hr 15 mins

Total: 1 hr 40 mins

Additional: 15 mins

Servings: 6

## Ingredients

1 (3 pound) of whole chicken, giblets removed

Salt and black pepper to taste

1 tablespoon of onion powder, or to taste

½ cup of margarine, divided

1 stalk of celery leaves removed

## Directions

Step 1

Preheat oven to 350 degrees F (175 degrees C).

Step 2

Place chicken in a roasting pan, and season generously inside and out with salt and pepper. Sprinkle inside and out with onion powder. Place 3 tablespoons margarine in the chicken cavity. Arrange dollops of the remaining margarine around the chicken's exterior. Cut the celery into 3 or 4 pieces, and place in the chicken cavity.

Step 3

Bake uncovered 1 hour and 15 minutes in the preheated oven, to a minimum internal temperature of 180 degrees F (82 degrees C). Remove from heat, and baste with melted margarine and drippings. Cover with aluminum foil, and allow to rest about 30 minutes before serving.

**Nutrition Facts**

Per Serving:

423 calories; 32.1 g total fat; 97 mg cholesterol; 662 mg sodium. 1.2 g carbohydrates; 30.9 g protein; Full Nutrition

## Spinach and Feta Pita Bake

**Recipe Summary**

Prep: 10 mins

Cook: 12 mins

Total: 22 mins

Servings: 6

**Ingredients**

1 (6 ounce) tub sun-dried tomato pesto

6 (6 inch) whole wheat pita breads

2 roma (plum) tomatoes, chopped

1 bunch of spinach, rinsed and chopped

4 fresh mushrooms, sliced

½ cup of crumbled feta cheese

2 tablespoons of grated Parmesan cheese

3 tablespoons of olive oil

Ground black pepper to taste

**Directions**

Step 1

Preheat the oven to 350 degrees F (175 degrees C).

Step 2

Spread tomato pesto onto one side of each pita bread and place them pesto-side up on a baking sheet. Top pitas with tomatoes, spinach, mushrooms, feta cheese, and Parmesan cheese; drizzle with olive oil and season with pepper.

Step 3

Bake in the preheated oven until pita breads are crisp, about 12 minutes. Cut pitas into quarters.

**Per Serving:**

350 calories; 17.1 g total fat; 13 mg cholesterol; 587 mg sodium. 41.6 g carbohydrates; 11.6 g protein; Full Nutrition

**Ingredients**

55 m

6 servings

273 cals

3 cloves garlic, minced 1/3 cup olive oil 1/4 cup tomato sauce 2 tablespoons red wine vinegar 2 tablespoons chopped fresh basil 1/2 teaspoon salt 1/4 teaspoon cayenne pepper 2 pounds fresh shrimp, peeled and deveined skewers

**Directions**

In a large bowl, stir together the garlic, olive oil, tomato sauce, and red wine vinegar. Season with basil, salt, and cayenne pepper. Add shrimp to the bowl, and stir until evenly coated. Cover, and refrigerate for 30 minutes to 1 hour, stirring once or twice.

Preheat grill for medium heat. Thread shrimp onto skewers, piercing once near the tail and once near the head. Discard marinade.

Lightly oil grill grate. Cook shrimp on preheated grill for 2 to 3 minutes per side, or until opaque.

Nutrition Facts

Per Serving: 273 calories; 14.7 g fat; 2.8 g carbohydrates; 31 g protein; 230 mg cholesterol; 472 mg sodium. Full nutrition

**Recipe Summary**

Prep: 5 mins

Cook: 5 hrs

Total: 5 hrs 5 mins

Servings: 6

**Ingredients**

1 (5 pound) of standing beef rib roast

2 teaspoons of salt

1 teaspoon of ground black pepper

1 teaspoon of garlic powder

**Directions**

Step 1

Allow roast to stand at room temperature for at least 1 hour.

Step 2

Preheat the oven to 375 degrees F (190 degrees C). Combine the salt, pepper and garlic powder in a small cup. Place the roast on a rack in a roasting pan so that the fatty side is up and the rib side is on the bottom. Rub the seasoning onto the roast.

Step 3

Roast for 1 hour in the preheated oven. Turn the oven off and leave the roast inside. Do not open the door. Leave it in there for 3 hours. 30 to 40 minutes before serving, turn the oven back on at 375 degrees F (190 degrees C) to reheat the roast. The internal temperature should be at least 145 degrees F (62 degrees C). Remove from the oven and let rest for 10 minutes before carving into servings.

**Nutrition Facts**

Per Serving:

576 calories; 46.2 g total fat; 137 mg cholesterol; 880 mg sodium. 0.6 g carbohydrates; 37 g protein; Full Nutrition

## Rosemary Roasted Turkey

**Ingredients**

4 h 45 m

16 servings

596 cals

3/4 cup olive oil 3 tablespoons minced garlic 2 tablespoons chopped fresh rosemary 1 tablespoon chopped fresh basil 1 tablespoon Italian seasoning 1 teaspoon ground black pepper salt to taste 1 (12 pound) whole turkey Add all ingredients to list

**Directions**

Preheat oven to 325 degrees F (165 degrees C).

In a small bowl, mix the olive oil, garlic, rosemary, basil, Italian seasoning, black pepper and salt. Set aside.

Wash the turkey inside and out; pat dry. Remove any large fat deposits. Loosen the skin from the breast. This is done by slowly working your fingers between the breast and the skin. Work it loose to the end of the drumstick, being careful not to tear the skin.

Using your hand, spread a generous amount of the rosemary mixture under the breast skin and down the thigh and leg. Rub the remainder of the rosemary mixture over the outside of the breast. Use toothpicks to seal skin over any exposed breast meat.

Place the turkey on a rack in a roasting pan. Add about 1/4 inch of water to the bottom of the pan. Roast in the preheated oven 3 to 4 hours, or until the internal temperature of the bird reaches 180 degrees F (80 degrees C).

**Nutrition Facts**

Per Serving: 596 calories; 33.7 g fat; 0.8 g carbohydrates; 68.1 g protein; 198 mg cholesterol; 165 mg sodium. Full nutrition

## Garlic Prime Rib

**Recipe Summary**

Prep: 10 mins

Cook: 1 hr 30 mins

Total: 1 hr 40 mins

Servings: 15

Yield: 1 - 10 pound roast

**Ingredients**

1 (10 pound) prime rib roast

10 cloves of garlic, minced

2 tablespoons of olive oil

2 teaspoons of salt

2 teaspoons of ground black pepper

2 teaspoons of dried thyme

**Directions**

Step 1

Place the roast in a roasting pan with the fatty side up. In a small bowl, mix together the garlic, olive oil, salt, pepper and thyme. Spread the mixture over the fatty layer of the roast, and let the roast sit out until it is at room temperature, no longer than 1 hour.

Step 2

Preheat the oven to 500 degrees F (260 degrees C).

Step 3

Bake the roast for 20 minutes in the preheated oven, then reduce the temperature to 325 degrees F (165 degrees C), and continue roasting for an additional 60 to 75 minutes. The internal temperature of the roast should be at 135 degrees F (57 degrees C) for medium rare.

Step 4

Allow the roast to rest for 10 or 15 minutes before carving so the meat can retain its juices.


**Nutrition Facts**

Per Serving:

562 calories; 48 g total fat; 113 mg cholesterol; 395 mg sodium. 1 g carbohydrates; 29.6 g protein; Full Nutrition

# Guacamole

Recipe Summary

Prep: 10 mins

Total: 10 mins

Servings: 4

**Ingredients**

3 avocados - peeled, pitted, and mashed

1 lime, juiced

1 teaspoon of salt

½ cup of diced onion

3 tablespoons of chopped fresh cilantro

2 roma (plum) tomatoes, diced

1 teaspoon of minced garlic

1 pinch of ground cayenne pepper (optional)

**Directions**

Step 1

In a medium bowl, mash together the avocados, lime juice, and salt. Mix in onion, cilantro, tomatoes, and garlic. Stir in cayenne pepper. Refrigerate 1 hour for best flavor, or serve immediately.

**Nutrition Facts**

Per Serving:

262 calories; 22.2 g total fat; 0 mg cholesterol; 596 mg sodium. 18 g carbohydrates; 3.7 g protein; Full Nutrition

## Taco Seasoning I

Ingredients

1 m

10 servings

5 cals

1 tablespoon of chili powder

1/4 teaspoon of garlic powder

1/4 teaspoon of onion powder

1/4 teaspoon of crushed red pepper flakes

1/4 teaspoon of dried oregano

1/2 teaspoon of paprika

1 1/2 teaspoons of ground cumin

1 teaspoon of sea salt

1 teaspoon of black pepper

Add all ingredients to list

**Directions**

Prep 1 m

Ready In 1 m

In a small bowl, mix together chili powder, garlic powder, onion powder, red pepper flakes, oregano, paprika, cumin, salt and pepper. Store in an airtight container.


**Nutrition Facts**

Per Serving: 5 calories; 0.2 g fat; 0.9 g carbohydrates; 0.2 g protein; 0 mg cholesterol; 185 mg sodium.


## Browning's Lymph Clear

**Ingredients**

**These are all added to POT#1**

1oz of Blood root Lymphatic. Showing results as an antibacterial and more. Showing great scientific promise in fighting cancers.

2oz of Burdock Root Lymphatic. Helps eliminate waste in the body, it is an antibiotic, antiseptic, and anti fungal, detoxifying herb.

2oz of Chaparral Lymphatic, plus it is an antibacterial, antiviral and anti-tumor.

1.5oz of Dandelion Root Liver and Pancreas filters and strains toxins.

1.5oz  of Echinacea Root Stimulates lymphatic activity and boosts immune system

2oz of Poke Root Lymphatic. The root has a very favorable influence on the glandular system.

2oz of Red Root It is an excellent lymphatic remedy. Stimulates lymph and tissue fluid circulation for drainage. Also effective on enlarged lymph nodes and for shrinking non fibrous cysts.

1.5oz of Sarsparilla Blood tonic. Especially good for removing heavy metals if taken properly. It contains calcium, copper, iron, iodine, manganese, potassium, silicon, sodium, sulfur, B-complex, and vitamins A, C and D.

2.5oz of Yellow Dock. It improves the function of the kidneys, liver, lymph glands, and intestines, thus aiding the body's natural cleansing processes. Has been used to help the body eliminate heavy metals including lead and arsenic.


**2 gallons Distilled Water**

**These are all added to POT #2**

1oz of Black Walnut effective for treating colitis, infections, liver, tuberculosis and tumors. Helps regulate blood sugar levels, burns excess toxins and fatty materials, rids the colon of parasites and contains magnesium which feeds the muscles and nerves. It has shown to have oxygenating abilities which kills parasites.

1oz of Celandine reported to exhibit anti-viral, anti-inflammatory and anti-tumor properties both in vitro and in vivo. It helps relieve inflammation and chronic disorders of the hepatic and biliary system and inflammation of the respiratory organs.

1oz of Cleavers One of the best tonics for the lymphatic system available. It treats swollen glands anywhere in the body and has been useful in the treatment of ulcers and tumors by lymphatic drainage which detoxifies the tissue. It is an alternative, helps remove obstructions and swelling. Helpful in clearing the urinary tract and kidneys.

2oz of Lemon Peel alkalizes the body and is excellent for liver and lymph.

1.5oz of Plantain Great for boosting the Immune system, combating infection, counters blood poisoning, removes toxins.

1.5oz of Red Clover Lymphatic. Clinical evidence shows that there is a basis for its long standing tradition in treating cancer.

16oz of Vegetable Glycerin

8-12oz of Black Strap Molasses

60oz of Raw Honey

4 Tbls of Citric Acid

1 large package of cheesecloth

Servings: 4

**Instructions**

Pot #1

Place ingredients in a large pot and set on a warm heat over night so roots may soften. In the morning, bring up the heat and simmer for about 4 hours. Then boil for 15-30 minutes. After boiling, remove from heat and strain the liquid into a clean container by placing a layer of cheesecloth over your strainer.

Pot #2

Cover and set on counter over night. In the morning, place the pot on warm /medium heat to steep NOT BOIL the herbs like you would a cup of tea. Let them steep for at least 4 hours then strain the liquid. These two steps can be done at the same time) Compost the strained herbs in your garden ( or give them to your chickens :-)) Once the liquid is strained form both pots, mix it together in one of the pots and let it simmer for about 15 minutes, then add 16 oz. vegetable glycerin, 8-12 oz Black Strap Molasses, 60 oz of Raw Honey, and 4

Tbls. Citric Acid. Stir and let the mixture mingle for about 15 minutes. When ready to bottle use a candy thermometer to check the temperature of the liquid. You want it to be at 190 degrees to prevent any bacteria from growing in the tonic. Maintain the heat temperature throughout the bottling. Be sure your jars are sterilized properly. Add tonic to hot jars, filling to 1/2 inch from the top of jar and cap. Let cool overnight. Check to make sure all jars have sealed properly and tonics can be stored for 1 year.

Recipe Notes

Once a jar has been opened you must refrigerate it. It will last for two months in the refrigerator. Sediment in the bottom is normal. Shake before using.

**Do not take if you are pregnant.**


**Dosage:**

Adult: 1 Tablespoon t time a day for prevention, 1 Tbls. 2 times a day for lymphoedema.  2 Tbls 2 times a day when breast and lymph is congested or cancerous.

- Distilled water

- Organic maple syrup

- Organic cayenne pepper

- Laxative tea (optional)

- Decaffeinated natural herbal tea (optional)

- Organic lemons

- Unrefined sea salt or Epsom salt (table salt will also work)

## Use natural fresh ingredients

Drinking pure filtered water or distilled water is considered among the best ways of cleansing your body naturally. For this reason, this ingredient is an crucial part of the master cleanse diet.

Avoid using tap water or bottled water as they contain chemicals that may be harmful to your health.

All the other ingredients should be organic. Non-organic fruits and vegetables are often sprayed with pesticides and other chemicals.

Avoid concentrated lemon juice as it is known to contain sugar and other preservatives. Also, you should only use Grade B maple syrup as processed syrup contains artificial flavors and high sugar concentration.

The syrup provides most of the calories. Hence the alternate name, "maple syrup diet".

The reason for using lemon and maple syrup is that they are a rich source of vitamins and minerals.

The sea salt should be unrefined. If you have issues with salt consumption, you should consider alternatives such as laxative tea. Table salt can be used if needed. However, the tea should not contain caffeine or any other elements that may hurt the effectiveness of the concoction.

## Master Cleanse Recipe: Serving information

- 12 Tablespoons of organic lime or lemon juice

- 12 Tablespoons of organic maple syrup

- 1/2 Teaspoon of cayenne pepper

- 60 ounces of pure filtered water

Above is our master cleanse recipe in a six serving recipe. Drink a minimum of 6 glasses of lemonade diet daily for best results.

Adding laxatives such as sea salt or herbal tea to your drink may help the detox process. They could also help rid excess fat faster. Remember to always consult a doctor first!

Experts recommend that you take this lemonade diet for about 10 days. This allows for safer, desirable results.


## Vegan Marbled Cake

This gorgeous cake needs no frosting in my opinion, as it offers plenty of sweet, sweet, goodness all by its lonesome. Plus, served undressed is the best way to show off its striking swirls.

Prep time:

20 minutes

Cook time:

35 minutes

Total time:

55 minutes


**Ingredients**

¾ cup of white rice flour

½ cup of brown rice flour

¾ cup of besan/chickpea flour

1 cup of potato starch

1½ of teaspoons xanthan gum

2½ of teaspoons baking powder

1 teaspoon of baking soda

1 cup of sugar

1 teaspoon of salt

¾ cup of olive oil

2 cups of very cold water

2 tablespoons of lemon juice

¼ cup of cocoa powder

**Instructions**

Preheat oven to 350°F. Lightly grease an 8 × 8-inch cake pan. In a large bowl, whisk together the rice flours, besan, potato starch, xanthan gum, baking powder, baking soda, sugar, and salt. Add the olive oil, water, and lemon juice and stir well to achieve a very smooth batter.

Pour about one-third of the batter into a bowl and whisk in the cocoa powder until evenly blended. Spread the yellow cake batter into the prepared baking pan and then drop dollops of the chocolate batter onto the yellow. Use a butter knife to gently swirl the two batters together into a loose and even pattern.

Bake the cake for 35 to 40 minutes, or until a knife inserted into the middle comes out clean. Let cool before slicing with a serrated knife. Store covered for up to 3 days.

**Nutrition Information**

Yield

10

Serving Size

1

Amount per Serving

Calories 424

Total Fat 17g

Saturated Fat 2g

Trans Fat 0g

Unsaturated Fat 14g

Cholesterol 0mg

Sodium 474mg

Carbohydrates 64g

Fiber 3g

Sugar 21g

Protein 5g

Japanese Beauty Hotpot BiJin Nabe（美人锅） – Collagen-rich Chicken Soup

Prep time:  1 hour

Cook time:  8 hours

Total time:  9 hours

Serves: 4 to 6 pax


**Ingredients**

**Pre-boiling the broth**

· 600g - 800g of Chicken Feet (or Wing Tip)

· 1500g of Chicken Bones

**Boiling the Broth**

· Cleaned and Scum-free Chicken Feet & Bones

· 6 Liters of water (Add more along the way - refer to post's body on when to add water)

**Finishing the Broth**

· 500ml Cooking Sake

· 2 tablespoon of Salt (please taste and adjust accordingly based on individual preference)

· 1 teaspoon of Sugar

· 6 pieces of Chicken Wings and Drumlette (Can be replaced with any parts of the chicken)

**Japanese Pork Tsukune**

· 250g of Minced Pork Belly (Can be replaced with minced pork or chicken)

· ½ tablespoon of cornstarch/ Potato Starch

· 1 teaspoon of Salt

· 1 tablespoon of Cooking Sake

· ¼ teaspoon of Grounded black pepper

· 1 egg

· 2 tablespoons of Cured Fish Roe (Tobiko)

**Suggested ingredients for hotpot**

· Golden Mushroom (Enoki)

· Baby Corn

· Soaked Black Fungus

· Mini Red Raddish

· Lettuce

· Prawns

· Bean curd Puff

· Pea sprout

· Noodles

· Rice

**Instructions**

**Pre Boiling the Bones & Feet**

1. Wash the feet (or tips) and bones and fill the pot with water until it fully covers the feet and bones. Let it boil under high heat for 5 minutes until all the scums of the feet and bones are floating on top of the pot of boiling water

2. Turn off the heat and remove the pot from the stove.

3. Pour away the water and its scum.

4. Wash and scrub the feets (or tips), bone and even pot. Ensure that not a single sight of the residues were remained

**Boiling the Broth**

1. Transfer the cleaned feet and bone back into the pot or any pot that can hold at least 6 liters of water.

2. Add in 6 litres of water to the pot of feets and bone; bring it to vigorous boil under medium high heat.

3. Once the pot of water is boiling, reduce the heat to medium (still boiling but not vigorously). Remove any floating scums if any.

4. Cover with lid, slightly ajar

5. Let it boil for about 8 hours or until the broth reached your desired milkiness and thickness (it will be slightly

sticky and thick due to the breakdown of collagen into the broth)

6. Add water occasionally to maintain a certain water level for boiling. *Refer to post content on how much water to add and when to add

**Finishing the broth**

1. When the broth reaches your desired thickness and milkiness, strained away all the bones and shreds of meat

2. The broth should be about 3 litres after straining.

3. Transfer the broth into a pot and allow it to boil over medium high heat

4. Add the chicken pieces (wings, drum, breast, thigh, etc) , seasoning and allow it to boil for 5 minutes

5. Allow it to cool before transferring to an airtight container or let it remain in the pot,

6. Transfer the pot or container or broth into the chiller and allow it to chill for at least 4 hours or overnight, until the broth set into pudding-like texture.

**Pork Belly Tsukune with Dynamite Crunch**

1. In a large mixing bowl, add in all the ingredients and seasoning.

2. Mix until well combine

3. Make it into balls, cling wrap it and chill it fridge until needed.

Assembling the Pot of Bijin Nabe

1. Sccop the pudding-like broth together with the chicken pieces into the pot for hotpot

2. Assemble the rest of the ingredients for the hotpot on a plate


## Watermelon Fries

**Ingredients:**

1 small watermelon, cut into fries

Zest from 1 lime

1 tbsp lime juice

1/2-1 tsp chili powder


**Directions:**

Arrange the watermelon fries on a plate or platter. Add the lime zest, juice and chili powder. Serve immediately.

Serves: 2


## Summer Cold Soup

**Directions**

Put all products in a blender/food processor and crush it to a paste like consistency. If the mass is too thick, you can add more buttermilk.

Taste and add salt, pepper or lemon juice to adjust. Best served with sprinkles of olive oil on top.

This delicious soup is meant to be served alone but as an option could be served with oven-baked potato slices (Phases 2 and 3).

Enjoy.


**Ingredients**

6 cucumbers

2 avocados

1/2 jalapeno

1 large clove garlic

Handful of fresh basil leaves

Handful of dill

5 sticks of scallions

1/2 lemon juice

20 oz buttermilk

3 tbsp of olive oil

2 tsp of apple vinegar

1 tsp of salt

1/4 tsp of pepper

Ceasar Salad Phase 3

**Directions**

To prepare the sauce, add all the ingredients for the sauce to the food grinder and crush it to paste like consistency.

To prepare the croutons, cut the bread into small cubes. In a bowl, mix the bread cubes with oil and spices, bake in a 390-degree oven for about 10 minutes, until the croutons are nicely scoffed and hardened.

Combine washed and well drained with avocado slices, crab sticks, croutons and parmesan cheese shavings.

Serve the sauce on the side to preserve the crispiness and freshness of the salad. Enjoy!

**Ingredients**

150g favorite salad leaves

1 large ripe avocado

1 tbsp of Lemon juice (can adjust to taste)

150g crab sticks

1/4 cup of Parmesan cheese

4 slices of white bread

2 tbsp of olive oil

Pinch of salt and pepper

**Sauce**

4 tbsp of mayonnaise

1 small clove garlic

2 anchovy fillets

1 tbsp of lemon juice

Splash of Worchester Sauce

Handful of grated parmesan

Pinch of salt and pepper


## Low calorie Omelette

**Directions**

Separate the eggs.

Add the milk to the egg whites and whisk together with a fork.

Spray the oil into a wide frying pan (skillet) and warm over a medium heat for at least 2 minutes.

Pour in the egg white mixture, then add the cherry tomatoes and basil immediately. Season with salt and pepper and cook until set. The omelette should cook in less than a minute. Serve straight away.

**Ingredients**

3 large eggs (54 cals for egg whites)

1 tbsp of skimmed milk

3 sprays light extra virgin olive oil

10 cherry tomatoes

Fresh basil leaves, torn (optional)

Salt & pepper to taste


**Nutrition Facts**

Calories84


## Grilled Salmon Kebabs

**Directions**

Begin by heating the grill to medium. Spray the grates with olive oil.

In a small bowl, mix the spices together. This includes the red pepper flakes, cumin, sesame seeds, and oregano. Set the mixture aside.

Next, take the salmon filets and cut it into 1 inch pieces. Take the lemons and slice them into very thin rounds.

Then you will grab the skewers (make sure they have been soaked) and beginning with the salmon thread the salmon chunk followed by a thin folded lemon slice. Thread the skewers so that salmon is at the beginning as well as the end of the skewer.

This should make 8 full skewers worth. Then spray the salmon with olive oil spray. Season the salmon the the spice mixture and a touch of salt.

Lastly, toss the kebabs onto the grill and allow cooking for about 8 to 10 minutes. Grill until the fish is opaque throughout. Make sure to turn occasionally to avoid burning. Enjoy!

**Ingredients**

2 Lemons

1 1/2 of lbs Wild Salmon Filets

2 tbsp of Fresh Oregano

2 tsp of Sesame Seeds

1 tsp of Ground Cumin

1/4 tsp of Crushed Red Pepper

1 tsp Salt

Olive Oil Cooking Spray

16 Bamboo Skewers (soaked for 1 hour)


Nutrition Facts

Serving Size2 Skewers

Calories267

**Directions**

Begin by preheating the oven to 400 degrees F.

Slice the squash into pieces and mix with the garlic, rosemary, olive oil, salt, and black pepper.

Line a baking sheet with parchment paper. Spread the squash mixture onto the baking sheet. Place the baking sheet in the oven to cook for about 45 to 50 minutes. Make sure that the squash is caramelized and golden brown in color before removing. Remove and enjoy!

**Ingredients**

1 Butternut Squash

2 Cloves of Garlic

2 Fresh Rosemary Sprigs

2 tbsp of Olive Oil

Sea Salt to Taste

Ground Black Pepper

**Directions**

Begin by preheating the oven to 425 degrees.

Cut the cauliflower head up into bite-sized florets. Toss the florets into a large baking dish with the oil, cumin, salt, and pepper. Mix well.

Next, Place the cauliflower in the oven to bake for about 30 minutes. Make sure to mix the ingredients around a couple of times throughout the outlined cook time to avoid certain areas being overcooked. While the cauliflower is baking, begin to de seed the pomegranate. It is best to do this in a bowl of water as it can get quite messy and the seeds are bound to fly every which way.

After about 25 minutes, remove the cauliflower if it has reached a point where it is tender and becoming golden in color. If this does not occur after that amount of time, go ahead and leave it in the oven to bake until it does.

Once fully roasted, remove the cauliflower and transfer it to serving dishes while it is still warm. You will then toss in the pomegranate seeds, mint, and greenery of your choice (if you feel like adding it). This dish tastes delicious without the additional greens as well. Enjoy!

**Ingredients**

1 Head of Cauliflower

2 tbsp of Extra-Virgin Olive Oil or Coconut Oil

1 tsp of Cumin

1 tsp of Salt

1/2 tsp of Pepper

1 Pomegranate

Chopped Fresh Mint Leaves

Optional Greens of Choice


## Homemade Apple Tea Recipe

**Directions**

Begin by placing the apple slices, cinnamon, cloves, and water in a saucepan. Bring to a boil.

Reduce the heat and allow the mixture to simmer for 15 minutes. Sweeten with honey or stevia, and strain into tea glasses. Push gently on the apples to remove all the liquid. Enjoy!

**Ingredients**

8 oz. Dried Apple Slices

2 Cinnamon Sticks

4 Cloves

1 1/2 quarts Cold Water

Honey or Stevia

## Warm Butternut Kale Quinoa Salad Cider Dijon Dressing

**Directions**

Begin by preheating the oven to 400 degrees.

Next, toss the cubed butternut squash in the oil, sugar, paprika, salt, coriander, cumin, black pepper, nutmeg, and cayenne pepper. Then take a rimmed sheet pan and spread the squah pieces evenly. Bake the squash for about 10 minutes, rotate the pan, and c o ntinue baking for another 10 minutes.

While the squash is in the oven, make the dressing. Combine the vinegars, mustard, honey, lemon juice, salt, and pepper in a glass jar. Add the oil last, secure the jar's lid and shake well.

Then place the chopped kale, cooked quinoa, roasted squash, raisins, dried cranberries, and pepitas in a large salad bowl. Use a pinch or two of kosher salt and freshly ground black pepper to season the salad.

Once the salad is prepared, drizzle with 1/4 cup of the dressing or more to taste. Serve warm. Enjoy!

**Ingredients**

For the squash:

4 cups of cubed butternut squash (1/2 inch pieces)

1 tablespoon of olive oil

1 tablespoon of dark brown sugar

1 teaspoon of smoked paprika

3/4 teaspoon of kosher salt

3/4 teaspoon of ground coriander

3/4 teaspoon of cumin

1/4 teaspoon of freshly ground black pepper

1/8 teaspoon of nutmeg

1/8 teaspoon of cayenne

**For the salad dressing:**

1 tablespoon of whole grain Dijon mustard

1/4 cup of cider vinegar

2 tablespoons of fresh lemon juice (strained to catch the seeds)

2 tablespoons of white wine vinegar

1/2 teaspoon of kosher salt

1/4 teaspoon of freshly ground black pepper

1/2 cup of olive oil

2 tablespoons of honey

**For the salad:**

1 bunch of lacinato kale, stripped off stems, rinsed and patted dry

4 cups of cooked quinoa (1 cup dry)

1/3 cup of roasted pumpkin (pepita) seeds

1/4 cup of dried cranberries

1/4 cup of golden raisins

Salt and pepper to taste


## Shrimp Plum Salad

**Directions**

Sauté shrimp on the stove top at medium-high with 1/2 tablespoon of olive oil, 1 forkful of minced garlic and pepper.

Put the remaining salad ingredients on a very large plate.

Whisk together salad dressing ingredients in a tiny bowl. This includes the mustard, 2 forkfuls of minced garlic, apple cider vinegar, and extra virgin olive oil

Top salad with shrimp and dressing! Enjoy.

**Ingredients**

7 Medium-Large Shrimp (One Serving)

1/2 tsp of Extra Virgin Olive Oil

3 Forkfuls of Minced Garlic from Jar

Fresh Ground Pepper

Large Plateful of Spring Mix Lettuce, with both green and red leaves

1/4 Sweet Onion, sliced

1/2 Cucumber, sliced

1 Plum, sliced

2 tbsp of Stone Ground Mustard

1/4 cup of Apple Cider Vinegar

1 tsp of Extra Virgin Olive Oil


## Spicy Shrimp Cilantro Lime

**Directions**

To make the seasoning, mix together the salt, paprika, cumin, curry powder, cayenne and cinnamon. Sprinkle over shrimp and toss to combine.

For grilling: Preheat your grill on medium heat and spray with cooking spray to prevent shrimp from sticking. Thread shrimp on skewers and place on grill for 1 to 2 minutes (until pink) then turn over and cook an additional 30 seconds to 1 minute, depending on how you like them. Squeeze lime juice over top and garnish with chopped cilantro, if desired.

For pan frying (add calories from olive oil): In a large skillet, heat 1 tablespoon of olive oil over medium-high heat. Add shrimp and cook, stirring occasionally for about 3 to 5 minutes. Shrimp should be opaque throughout. Squeeze lime juice over top and garnish with chopped cilantro, if desired. Enjoy!

**Ingredients**

2 lbs of large shrimp, deveined

3/4 tsp of salt

1 tsp of paprika

1/2 tsp of ground cumin

1/2 tsp of curry powder

1/8 tsp of cayenne pepper

1/8 tsp of cinnamon

Garnish with chopped cilantro and lime wedges

## CONCLUSION

There is no special diet for lymphedema. An accepted nutritional approach in the management of lymphedema is to follow a balanced diet, which in addition to physical activity and exercises promotes weight loss. Excessive weight contributes to greater demands on the lymphatic systems ability to drain fluid from the tissues; weight control therefore positively affects lymphedema.

Studies indicate that obesity does have an influence on lymph fluid level and extremity volume. Obesity and overweight often worsen the symptoms associated with lymphedema; a nutrition balanced and portion appropriate diet contributes in reducing the risk factors associated with lymphedema.

A balanced healthy diet including whole grains, fish, fruits and vegetables and avoiding fatty foods will greatly assist in achieving and maintaining a healthy weight without restricting the intake of important nutrients and vitamins. Crash diets or diets which restrict certain food groups and nutrients are not advisable.

There is a common misconception that lymphedema may be positively affected by limiting the protein intake. This is not the case although lymphedema is defined as an accumulation of water and protein in the tissues, it is essential to understand that lymphedema cannot be reduced by the limitation of protein ingestion, which can even be potentially dangerous. It is also important not to limit fluid intake in an attempt to reduce the swelling. Good hydration (water) is essential for basic cell function and esp e c i a lly important before and after lymphedema treatment to assist the body in eliminating waste products.

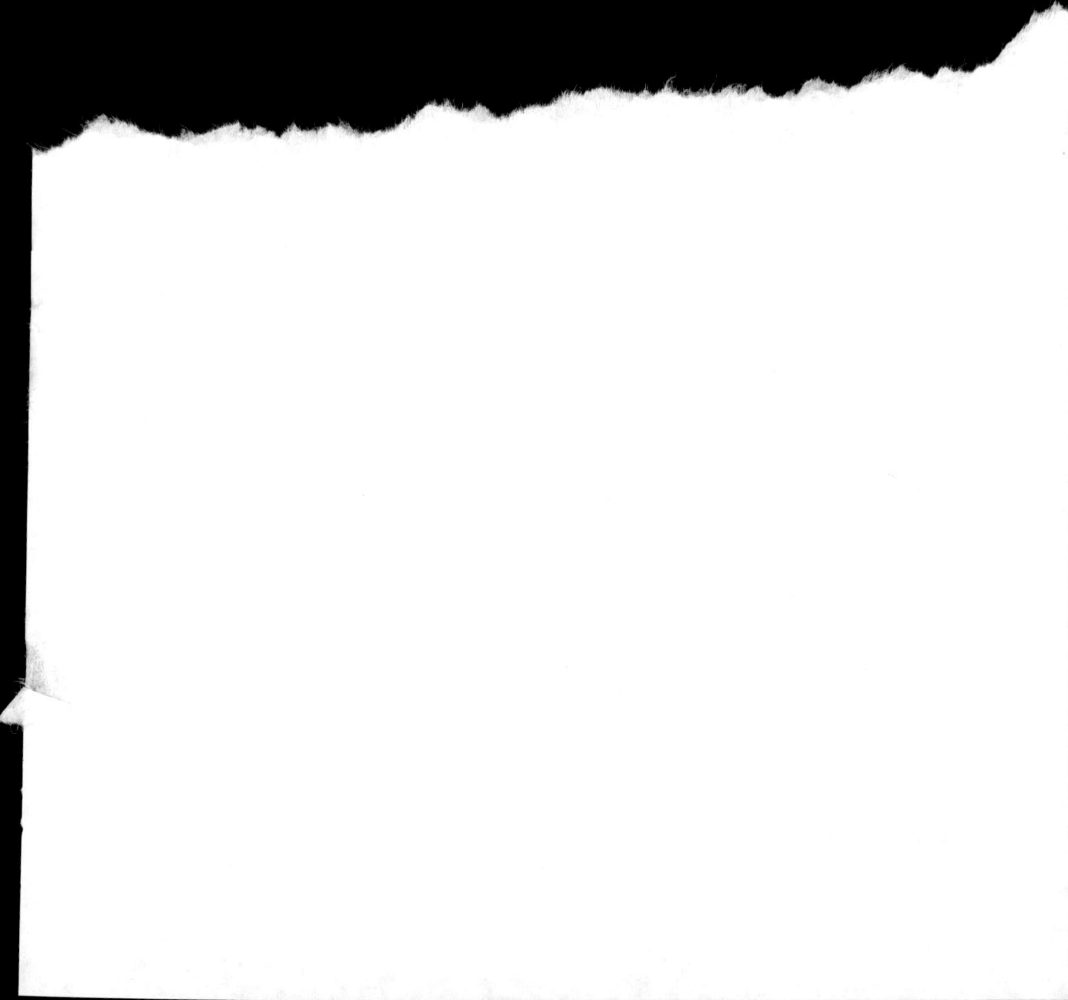

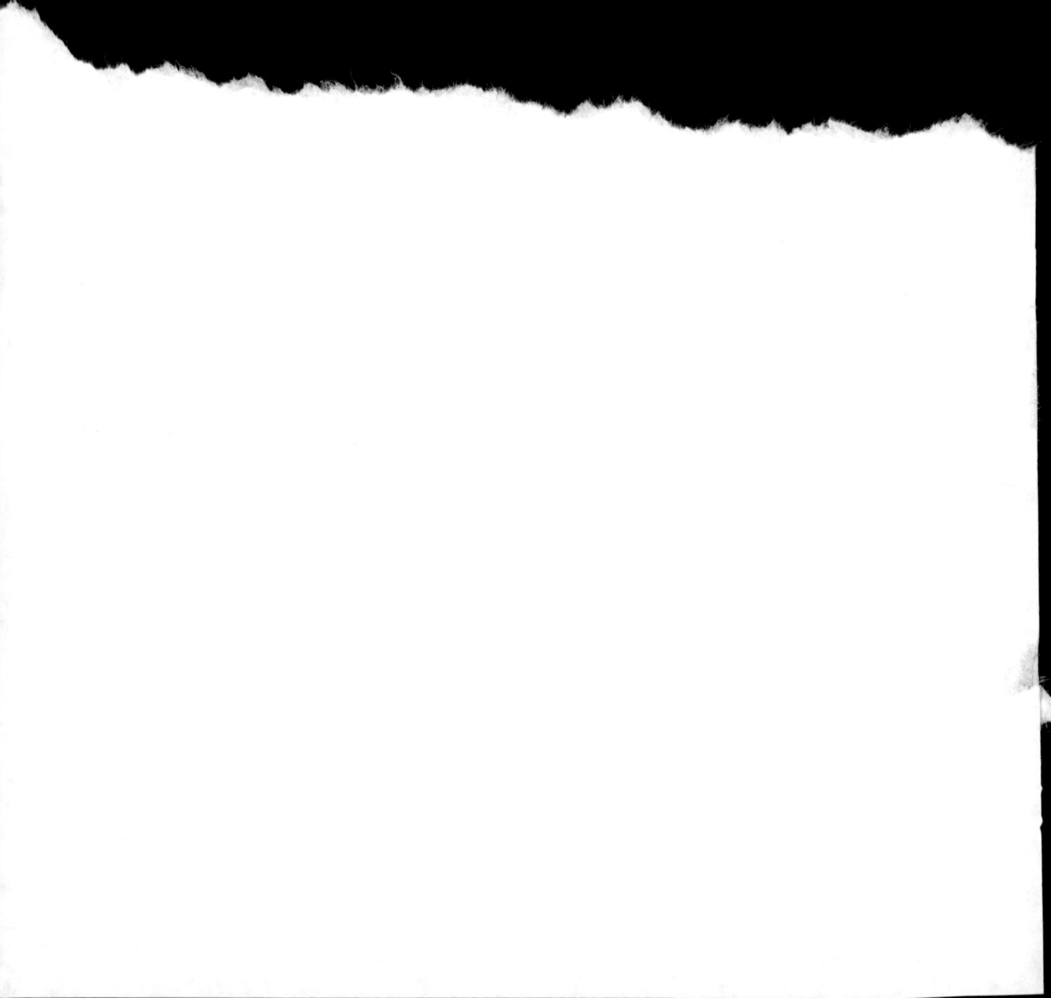